Learning

Reiki

is

Easy

MA Rivera

Editing: Tamara Beach
Cover Art: MA Rivera and Susan Beach
ISBN: 978-1-7363755-0-1
Library of Congress Control Number: 2021900151

Advance Praise

"MA Rivera is a gifted Reiki practitioner who has been tapped by angels to spread the love that is Reiki far and wide in the world through the release of *Learning Reiki Is Easy*. Ms. Rivera's book introduces readers to messages and instructions from Archangels and Ascended Masters while presenting additional information including non-traditional Reiki symbols to those who are studying Reiki with a Reiki Master Teacher."

~ Raven Keyes, MRMT, RMT, author of *The Healing Power of Reiki* and *The Healing Light of Angels*

"MA Rivera's love and healing energy touch every page of *Learning Reiki Is Easy*. Her information is clear and simple, and perfect for both the new Reiki practitioner as well as established practitioners who are looking for more guidance. Her detailed information on the Archangels is an added benefit to any healer. This book is a true gift."

~ Randi Botnick, Psychic Healer and Spiritual Counselor, and author of *4th-Dimensional Healing: A Guidebook for a New Paradigm of Healing*

TO HUMANITY IN
FAITH, HOPE, & LOVE

Contents

Introduction i

One: Universal Energy 1

Two: The Subtle Energy Body 5

Three: How to Do Reiki 9

Four: Reiki Symbols 15

Five: Self-Reiki 29

Six: Giving Reiki to Loved Ones 41

Seven: Archangels 51

Eight: Meet the Archangels 53

Nine: Attunement 79

Ten: Petition for Attunement 81

Eleven: Give Five 83

Twelve: Recommended Resources 85

About the Author 87

Acknowledgments

In Gratitude

First, I would like to thank my family and friends who supported me as I worked diligently in a crazily tight schedule to write this book to get it published in December 2020.

I would like to give thanks to Tamara Beach, who proofread and edited the final draft in such a tight schedule. Thank you so much. I truly appreciate your support.

I would like to give special thanks to Kala Ambrose, who helped me get started in the path for the creation of this book. Thank you so much. I truly appreciate your support.

I would like to give special thanks to Raven Keyes, who gave me feedback about the book. Thank you so much. I truly appreciate your support.

I have had the blessing of learning from many great teachers, for which I am very grateful. Many thanks to all my teachers, including but not limited to, Kala Ambrose, Julianne Bien, Randi Botnick, Dolores Cannon, Julia Cannon, Donna Eden, Richard Gordon, Heather Hildebrand, Doreya Karim, Laila Karim, Raven Keyes, Madison King, Katalin Koda, Tricia

McCannon, Grandmother Mechi, William Lee Rand, Carla Rueckert, Maruti Seidman, and Radleigh Valentine.

Last but not least, I would also like to give special thanks to my guardian angels, and all my guides and teachers in the spiritual realm that have helped me so much throughout the years. I would not be where I am now without their support. Many thanks to my guardian angels, and all my guides and teachers, including Yin, Yang, Felicidad, Obedience, Bartholomew, Cobalt, Archangel Michael, Jesus Christ, Lao Tzu, Lord Lanto, Master Adama, and Ascended Master John the Beloved.

Tribute

The creation of this book was made possible through the support of the Angelic Host, Ascended Masters, Master Adama, and other beings of Love and Light.

Especially, this book was made possible by the Archangels and a group of Ascended Masters who were very supportive and kept a constant presence while I was working on this book. I consider them to be the *Learning Reiki is Easy* Team of Love & Light.

***Learning Reiki is Easy* Team of Love & Light**

<u>Archangels</u>:

Ariel	Michael
Azrael	Raguel
Chamuel	Raphael
Gabriel	Raziel
Haniel	Sandalphon
Jeremiel	Uriel
Jophiel	Uzziel
Metatron	Zadkiel

<u>Ascended Masters</u>:

Lord Lanto

John the Beloved

El Morya

Lord Sananda

Lady Nada

Lao Tzu

Buddha Gautama

St. Germain

I am forever grateful for your assistance.
Thank you. Thank you. Thank you.

Message from Ascended Master John the Beloved

Grand Tetons
August 31, 2020

Dear Beloved,

It is with great joy and love that the Angelic Host, Ascended Masters, and other beings of Love and Light have put plans in motion for this long-awaited message to reach humanity.

We made contact, and she faithfully agreed to be of service as the scribe for the words to take form in the material and reach humanity. She had knowledge of the matter of connecting with the Universal Energy and had supported the activities of the Light in the past.

For the Universal Energy is ever-present; it is critical for humanity to reestablish connection to successfully and gracefully endeavor in the transit ahead, as this connection will illuminate those activities to reach full potential.

Humanity is in a critical time, for these are times of turmoil. But keep faith that these are most needed since they lead to the break and rearrangement of many facets of current civilization to make way to the bright future of humanity.

Blessings in Love and Light,
Ascended Master John the Beloved

A Message from the Heart

Grand Tetons, August 2020

About two months ago, I was contacted by Lord Lanto and shown the Grand Tetons. I arrived at the Grand Tetons in faith, hope and love, following the guidance of loving beings in service to the Light who are supporting humankind's evolution.

While driving down the Grand Tetons National Park, I felt the reach of the energies of the mountains and immediately knew that that the energies would help the creation of this book and that it would be a life-changing experience.

So, let me tell you how I found Reiki. My background is in hard science. During the late summer of 2010, I was reading about stones and crystals, as I have always been attracted to them. I was searching for a particular book on the internet when I stumbled across the announcement of an upcoming Reiki class on the main web page of the metaphysical store that was selling a used copy of the book I wanted. I read the announcement and felt a compelling urge coming from deep within my heart that I needed to be in that class. I could not ignore it. Prior to that time, I thought that Reiki was baloney. Oh boy, was I in for a surprise! ☺

After taking the Reiki class, I could feel the energy in my hands, and I could not deny that it was real. I realized then that Reality was much more than what I was taught in school and college.

I had awakened. My life has never been the same—thankfully. Hope this book does the same for you.

Love & Light,
MA Rivera

May the energies of Jupiter propel this book forward to a glorious success.
For this book is a gift from the loving beings in service to the Light.
Humanity, it is time to wake up!

Introduction

The purpose of this book is for humanity to reconnect consciously with the Universal Energy that the great Usui Sensei called Reiki. This connection is so important during this critical time in history when humanity is facing the COVID-19 pandemic. Hopefully, this reconnection also becomes a catalyst in raising human consciousness.

By means of a special dispensation, several Archangels have lovingly agreed to provide attunements. After reading this book completely, the person can petition for an attunement by an Archangel. The attunement will reconnect the person with the Universal Energy, and the person will be able to do Reiki for self and loved ones.

IF FOLLOWING, THE PERSON FEELS THE CALLING <u>TO BECOME A REIKI PRACTITIONER</u>, THE ANGELS RECOMMEND AND THE ACCEPTED PRACTICE IS FOR THE PERSON TO <u>STUDY UNDER A REIKI MASTER TEACHER AND BECOME CERTIFIED</u>.

Concerning how to write this book, I was instructed by Ascended Master John the Beloved to keep it simple, short, and sweet as well as easy to read and easy to follow. So, I tried my best to write in a brief and simple manner and provided recommendations for those seeking further information.

This book is homemade. It was created with much love during the COVID-19 pandemic. The energies from the loving beings in service to the Light permeate this book. So, do not be fooled by its simple manner. It truly is the real deal. Heed the warning.

<u>WARNING</u>
WRITTEN UNDER DIVINE INFLUENCE.
THIS BOOK MAY CHANGE YOUR LIFE.

One
Universal Energy

From my heavenly teachers, I learned that the Universal Energy is everywhere. It is important to understand that everything is energy. Energy can be in different frequencies/vibrational levels and have different functions; but when everything is said and done, energy is everything.

I also learned from my heavenly teachers that humanity was consciously connected to the Universal Energy before The Fall. People remembered who they were and knew how to use the Universal Energy. Those who felt the calling to be of service to others as healers would become apprentices at the healing temples. They would be carefully mentored by a teacher so they could specialize as healers and thus be able to give treatments at the healing temples. The Fall was truly a fall in human consciousness. Most of humanity became disconnected from the Universal Energy and forgot who they were.

The Resurfacing of Reiki
I will briefly cover the resurfacing of Reiki and its movement to the Western world as it was taught to me. I have had the blessing of learning Reiki from

1

several Reiki Master Teachers, including Raven Keyes, Katalin Koda, and William Lee Rand.

I was taught that Reiki supports stress reduction, relaxation, and healing. Reiki is composed of the two Japanese words/characters: Rei (Universal) and Ki (Life Energy), which commonly translates to "Universal Life Energy." I will use "Universal Energy" for short.

I was taught that Mr. Mikao Usui, for whom I will use the honorific Usui Sensei, connected with the Universal Energy while in deep meditation at Mount Kurama. Afterward, Usui Sensei, in great generosity and service to others, traveled throughout Japan giving Reiki treatments and teaching Reiki to many people.

I was taught that Dr. Chujiro Hayashi learned Reiki directly from Usui Sensei. Hayashi Sensei, in great generosity and service to others, had a clinic where free Reiki treatments were provided and taught Reiki to many people.

I was taught that Mrs. Hawayo Takata learned Reiki directly from Hayashi Sensei. Reiki made it to the Western world thanks to Takata Sensei. She gave Reiki treatments in Hawaii. Later in life, Takata Sensei taught Reiki to a set number of students who became Reiki Master Teachers under her, and through them,

Reiki spread throughout the United States and from there to other parts of the world.

The Angels convey great gratitude and blessings to Usui Sensei and his students, and their students and so on, for their support in raising the awareness of Reiki in the world.

For more information concerning Reiki, I recommend:

The Healing Power of Reiki by Raven Keyes

Sacred Path of Reiki: Healing as a Spiritual Discipline by Katalin Koda

Reiki Fire: New Information About the Origins of the Reiki Power: A Complete Manual by Frank Arjava Petter

Reiki: The Healing Touch: First and Second Degree Manual by William Lee Rand

Two
The Subtle Energy Body

The subtle energy body is composed of several energy systems including the aura, meridians, and chakras. I will briefly cover the aura, meridians, and the traditional seven-chakra system as they were taught to me. In addition to my Reiki Master Teachers, I have had the blessing of learning about the subtle energy body from several teachers, including Kala Ambrose, Donna Eden, Richard Gordon, and Maruti Seidman.

The Aura
The aura completely surrounds the body. It provides protection from the harsh energies in the environment around you. It is like your personal energetic spacesuit. The aura also selectively facilitates the movement of energy and information from the environment around you to the chakras and meridians, and from the chakras and meridians back out to the environment. The aura is composed of several layers, including the etheric, mental, and emotional layers.

Meridians
Meridians are like rivers of energy that flow through certain pathways to help nurture and replenish the body. There are 12 meridians plus the conception vessel and the governing vessel. Kidney and bladder

meridians are the primary grounding meridians. The kidney meridian takes energy into the body through the soles of the feet and moves it up the body while the bladder meridian moves the energy down the body and takes it out through the little toes. Walking barefoot on grass is one thing that helps with grounding.

Chakras
There are several energy centers on the body. These energy centers are also called chakras. These energy centers hold, move, and process energy; hold information; and interact with other energy systems to help nurture and replenish the body.

There are several main chakras located at certain points on the midline of the body. There are also several secondary chakras throughout the body, including the hands and feet. There is a chakra on the palm of each hand. Also, there is a chakra on the sole of each foot.

The traditional seven-chakra system is covered below, including other known chakra names and basic locations.

First Chakra	Root Chakra	Base of Spine
Second Chakra	Sacral Chakra	Lower Abdomen
Third Chakra	Power Chakra	Solar Plexus
Fourth Chakra	Heart Chakra	Heart
Fifth Chakra	Throat Chakra	Throat
Sixth Chakra	Third Eye Chakra	Forehead
Seventh Chakra	Crown Chakra	Top of Head

For more information on the subtle energy body, I recommend:

The Awakened Aura by Kala Ambrose

The Subtle Energy: An Encyclopedia of Your Energetic Anatomy by Cyndi Dale

Energy Medicine by Donna Eden

Balancing the Chakras by Maruti Seidman

Three
How to Do Reiki

Steps on how to do self-Reiki and giving Reiki to your loved ones will be covered in the following sections. General guidance will be covered first, then the descriptions of the Reiki symbols, followed by how to do self-Reiki and ending with giving Reiki to your loved ones.

GENERAL GUIDANCE
Be Comfortable
Get in a comfortable position, sitting on a chair or lying on your back (i.e., on the sofa) for doing self-Reiki. I like to do self-Reiki while lying on my back on the bed before going to sleep. After working on my desk for a while, I also like to take a quick break and do self-Reiki. I find Reiki to be very relaxing.

When giving Reiki to your loved ones, make sure that both of you are comfortable and keep soft lighting. Playing soft music is nice but optional.

The person giving Reiki can be kneeling on a pillow/cushion, sitting on a chair, or standing, depending on the area where Reiki is being given and the position of the person receiving Reiki.

The person receiving Reiki is usually lying on their back with their eyes closed to maximize relaxation. If the area needing attention is the back, the person receiving Reiki can be lying on their stomach or on one side—whichever is more comfortable. If the area needing attention is the head or shoulders, the person receiving Reiki can be sitting on a chair.

Remember to have a blanket close by because people tend to get cold when they relax.

Do-Nots
When giving Reiki to others, <u>do not touch sensitive areas,</u> including neck, face, breasts, and groin. If the neck or face areas need attention, give Reiki while maintaining hands in the air about six inches above the surface. If the breast, lower abdomen, or sacrum areas need attention, give Reiki while maintaining hands in the air about 18 inches above the surface.

When giving Reiki to others, <u>do not touch painful areas</u>. Before giving Reiki, remember to ask if there are any painful areas in the body. For painful areas, give Reiki while maintaining hands in the air about six inches above the surface.

If the person receiving Reiki is lying on the floor, <u>do not step over the person</u>; go around the person when changing positions.

Relaxed Hands

When doing Reiki, maintain relaxed hands (just slightly cupped) while keeping fingers together. The palms of the hands face the area you are sending Reiki. Having the hands just slightly cupped makes it easier for the fingers to stay together and for the hands to stay relaxed. If a finger tends to separate a little (i.e., pinky or thumb, which happens to me ☺), that's okay. The key is to be relaxed.

Centering and Setting Intention

While taking deep breaths and letting them out, do the following to help center yourself and set the intention before doing Reiki:

---Rub your hands together for a few seconds and then shake them off

---Place your hands on the front of your thighs and imagine roots coming from your feet going deep inside Mother Earth (do this for a few breaths)

---Raise your hands to the heart level and put them in prayer position

---Still your mind and while focusing on your heart, say out loud (or in your mind) a prayer or affirmation and set the intention that Reiki (Universal Energy) is moving through your hands and wait until you feel that you are ready to start doing Reiki.

Tracing Infinity/8

Energy can accumulate in areas of the body, such as body joints, becoming stagnant; eventually, the area gets very congested. Tracing the infinity symbol (∞) or the number 8 over the body helps move the energy and clear areas where energy is congested.

Tracing 8s on joints (such as knees, wrists, etc.) can help the flow of energy in those areas. Also, I find that tracing a few big 8s in the air about 18 inches above the person receiving Reiki is a good finishing move when giving a Reiki session. Trace a few big 8s with your hands about eight to 12 inches above the torso for self-Reiki. I feel that it helps sweep away any remaining stagnant energies over the body.

Connecting Heart and Solar Plexus
This is nice for completing self-Reiki, and it works by itself as well.
Place one hand on top of the other on the center of the chest on the heart area.
Take deep breaths and still your mind, and while focusing on your heart, you can say out loud (or in your mind) a prayer or affirmation.
Next, move the top hand to the solar plexus area while keeping the other hand on the heart area.
Hold for as long as you like.

Reiki Hand Positions
Several hand positions for self-Reiki and giving Reiki to your loved ones are covered in this book. These hand positions are recommendations; they are not set in stone. So, feel free to use them if you like them

or go ahead and experiment with hand positions that you like better. The key is for you to use the hand positions that you feel are working for you.

You can give Reiki by placing the hands directly on the body, or you can give Reiki while maintaining hands in the air about one or two inches above the surface.

Remember:
---Be comfortable
---Center yourself and set the intention
---Relaxed hands

Four
Reiki Symbols

The Angels ask for you to remember that you create your reality. So, say to yourself:

I manifest everything in my life.
I take responsibility for my life.
I have the power to change my life.

The creation process is influenced by your actions, beliefs, thoughts, and emotions; in turn, your actions and beliefs are also influenced by your thoughts and emotions. That is why it is so important to pay attention to your thoughts and emotions and keep them positive.

As you live your life and face challenges and setbacks, work diligently to bring in positive thoughts and emotions and stay in balance. Remember to call upon the Angels to help you stay positive and upbeat. Give all your worries, fears, and concerns to the Angels.

The Angels have provided several Reiki symbols to help humanity. They will help you create a reality infused with positive thoughts and emotions.

Let's together co-create a beautiful
future for humanity.

15

Reiki symbols act as facilitators to a function/attribute. You can think, visualize, trace with your finger/hand, or draw the symbols to use them. The different Reiki symbols will be covered in this section.

Power

The Power symbol has four main uses:

---to increase the strength of Reiki

---to focus Reiki on a particular area of the body or location

---for sealing and protection

---as a booster to the other symbols

The Power symbol is a very energetic symbol that resembles a musical treble clef. The Power symbol starts at the lower end and does a half loop, then moves upward in a direct line and then does a reversed half loop, and then it spirals in.

Examples:

While you are giving Reiki, you can think of or visualize the symbol to increase the strength of Reiki.

You can use the Power symbol on any area of the body that you feel needs extra Reiki.

As a booster, you can use a Reiki symbol (i.e., the Joy symbol) and follow with the Power symbol.

Before self-Reiki or giving Reiki, I like to trace the Power symbol on my palms to increase the strength of Reiki.

Before giving Reiki, I prepare the room by tracing in the air the Clearing symbol followed by the Power symbol on all the walls, ceiling, center of room, and floor. Following that, I trace a big Power symbol on my torso.

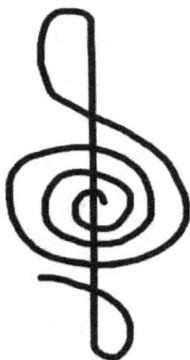

Power

Clearing

The Clearing symbol has several uses:

---to help clear the body of stagnant or blocked energies

---to clear away mental and emotional blockages

---to clear away habits and ways of thinking that no longer serve you

---to clear objects and living spaces

---to help to go through highly mental and/or emotional activities or situations

The Clearing symbol reminds me of the movement of water because it resembles waves/ripples. The Clearing symbol starts on the left and does an upward loop, then a downward loop and so on (total of three upward loops and two downward loops). When drawing/tracing the Clearing symbol, the shape of the loops does not need to be exact.

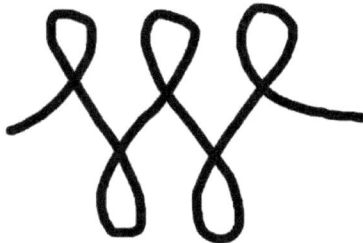

Clearing

Time/Space

The Time/Space symbol allows for Reiki to be sent to anywhere in the world and at any time (past, present, and future).

The Time/Space symbol starts with a circle at the top, then a horizontal line below, then a short vertical line connecting the circle and horizontal line. An infinity symbol follows below.

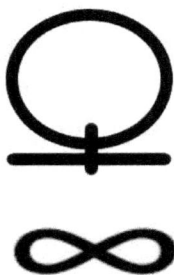

Time/Space

Among the first lessons that I received from my heavenly teachers was that Time/Space is irrelevant. All is in the here and now. We are all one. Separation is an illusion. Time is an illusion.

When you practice using this symbol to send distance Reiki, you can send Reiki to Mother Earth, to humanity, to the oceans, to the forests, etc...

When sending distance Reiki to a person, ask for permission from the person beforehand. If circumstances do not allow for getting permission beforehand (i.e., person is unconscious after an accident), then you can send distance Reiki by saying out loud (or in your mind) beforehand the following:

"With much love, I am sending
Reiki to (person's name).
May the Reiki reach (person's name) with the
permission of their Higher Self.
Otherwise, may the Reiki go where it
can be for the highest good."

Faith

The Faith symbol helps to boost your faith. It resembles the outline of mountains with an arrow pointing to the right to show movement. The Faith symbol is based on the proverb *"Faith can move mountains"* (Matthew 17:20).

When drawing/tracing the Faith symbol, the shape of the mountains does not need to be exact. Just set the intention that it resembles mountains.

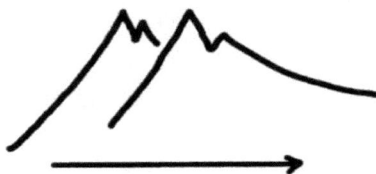

Faith

Hope

The Hope symbol helps to boost your hope. It resembles the Sun. It is based on the belief that the Sun brings a new day full of hope. There are many related sayings in current society, such as: *"Tomorrow is another day," "Tomorrow is a new day," "The Sun will shine tomorrow,"* and *"The Sun will come out tomorrow."*

I was shown two versions: the spiral Sun and the happy face Sun. Both work, so it is your choice which one you want to use when you are using it. I like them both, so I alternate when I'm using it.

When drawing/tracing the Hope symbol, it is a circle surrounded by lines with a happy face or a spiral inside. The shape of the Sun or the shape of the rays or the number of rays or the number of loops in the spiral do not need to be exact. Just set the intention when drawing/tracing the Hope symbol that it resembles a spiral Sun or a happy face Sun, whichever you are using.

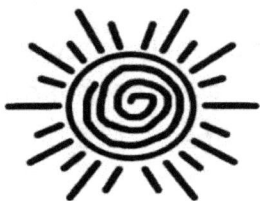

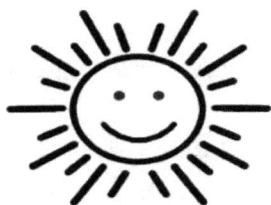

Hope

Love

The Love symbol helps to boost your love for yourself and others. It is a very energetic symbol that resembles a heart-shaped musical note. It will help bring love in its many manifestations into your life. The Love symbol will help attract what makes your heart sing.

The Love symbol starts on the left and does an upward loop, then a downward loop, and then goes up to end in a spiral. When drawing/tracing the Love symbol, the shape of the loops and the shape of the spiral do not need to be exact.

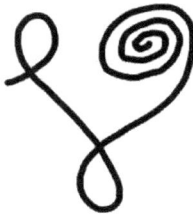

Love

Joy

The Joy symbol helps to boost your joy of life and attracts things that bring joy into your life. The Joy symbol resembles a butterfly. The butterfly is a symbol of joy, transformation, and evolution. The Joy symbol will help to bring out your inner child, who will remind you of the joy of watching butterflies fly by.

When drawing/tracing the Joy symbol, the shape of the wings or the trunk or the antennas do not need to be exact. Just set the intention that it resembles a butterfly.

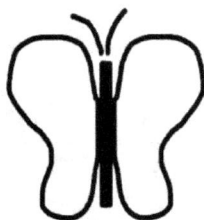

Joy

Happiness

The Happiness symbol helps to boost your happiness and attracts things that bring happiness into your life. The Happiness symbol resembles a sunflower. The sunflower is a symbol of happiness, love, and joy.

As the sunflowers faithfully face the Sun,
May you lovingly gaze at the Great Central Sun.

I was shown two versions: the spiral sunflower and the happy face sunflower. Both work, so it is your choice which one you want to use when you are using it. I like them both, so I alternate when I'm using it.

When drawing/tracing the Happiness symbol, it is a circle surrounded by petals with a happy face or a spiral inside and a vertical line for a stalk with two leaves. The shape of the sunflower (i.e., circle, petals, spiral) or the number of petals do not need to be exact. Just set the intention when drawing/tracing the Happiness symbol that it resembles a spiral sunflower or a happy face sunflower, whichever you are using.

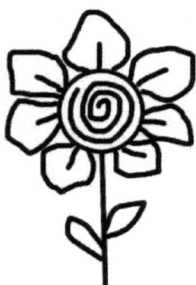

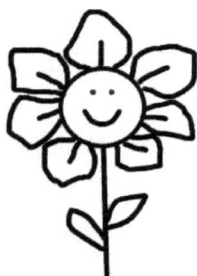

Happiness

Five
Self-Reiki

You can do self-Reiki as often as you want, whenever you can, and for as long as you like. Self-Reiki can be done on a daily basis during morning, day, or night, which will take anywhere from 15 minutes to one hour—your choice. Following are several recommended hand positions for self-Reiki.

Remember:
---Be comfortable
---Center yourself and set the intention
---Relaxed hands
---Use the Reiki symbols as you feel guided

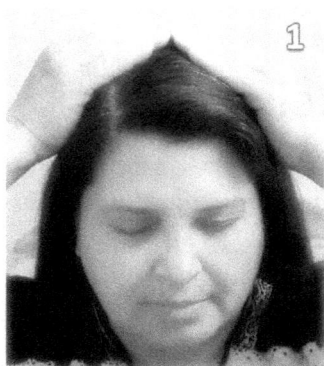
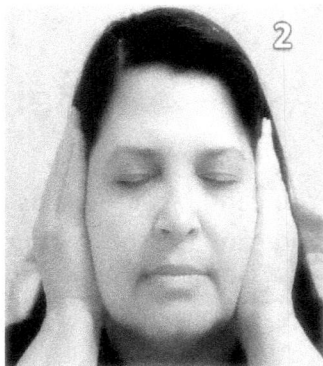
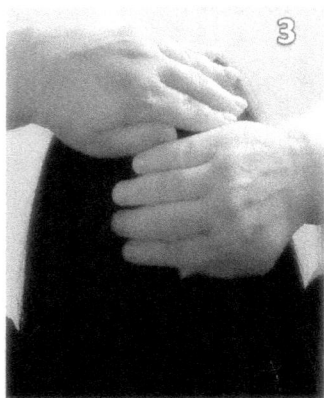
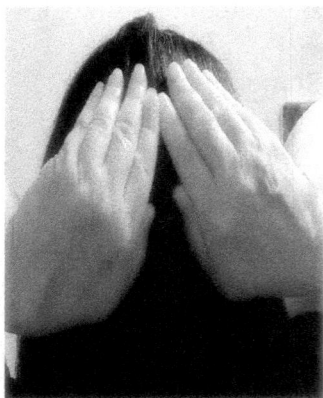
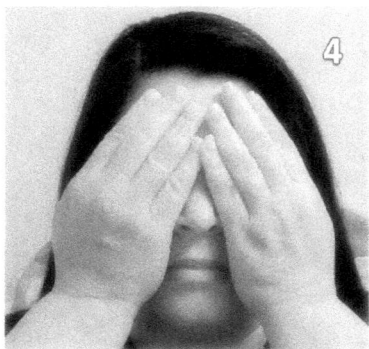

HEAD

1. Top of Head: Place your hands on top of the head with fingertips touching at the middle of the crown.

2. Sides of Head: Then, slide the hands down to cover the ears. The thumb side of the hand would be resting back toward the ears on the end of the jaw.

If you are lying down or reaching the back of your head is difficult, you can stay longer on the sides-of-the-head position and skip the back-of-the-head position.

3. Back of Head: You can either place the hands on the back of the head sideways (with fingertips pointing to the sides of the head) or both hands upward (with fingertips pointing to the top of the head).

4. Face: Gently place the hands on the face (covering the forehead, eyes, and cheeks while keeping the nose area open).

5. Jaw: Cover the mouth and jaw by placing the hands with the bottom of the palms touching in line with the tip of the chin. Alternative: it can also be done one side of the jaw at a time by placing one hand on the opposite side of the jaw and then switching sides with the other hand.

6. Neck: Then, slide the hands down to cover the neck gently. Alternative: it can also be done one side of the neck at a time by placing one hand on the opposite side of the neck and then switching sides with the other hand.

7. Shoulders: Place hands on the shoulders. I prefer to do this by crossing the arms and placing each hand on the opposite shoulder. Alternative: it can also be done one shoulder at a time by placing one hand on the opposite shoulder and then switching sides with the other hand.

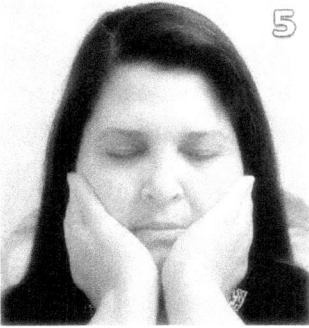
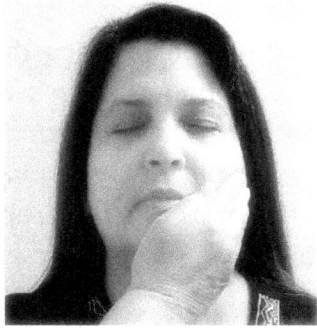

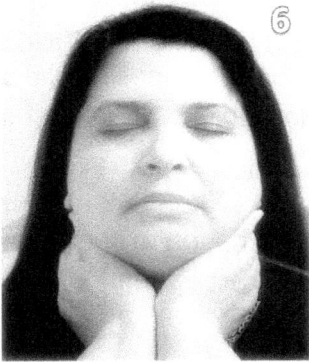
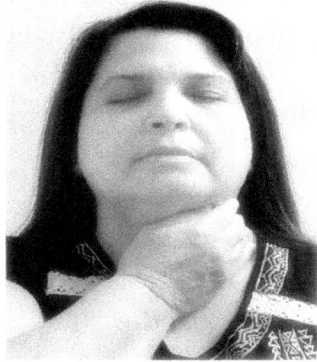

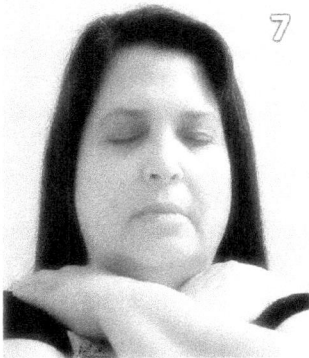
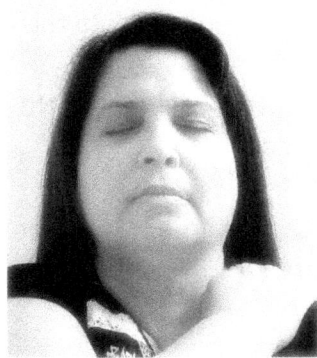

TORSO

You will be covering the torso by sliding the hands down about a palm's width at a time. Place hands with the fingertips touching (at the centerline of the torso) but not intertwined. It is okay to place the hands with the fingertips at a close distance but not touching; the key is to be comfortable.

8. Clavicle (Collarbone): Place hands on the clavicle on the upper torso area. This helps with grounding. If you prefer, it can also be done one side of the clavicle at a time by placing one hand on the opposite side of the clavicle and then switching sides with the other hand.

9. Upper Chest: Slide down the hands to the upper chest area. This sends energy to the lungs and the thymus gland.

10. Breast: Slide the hands down to the breast area. This is nurturing to the heart and the inner child.

11. Rib Cage: Slide the hands down to the rib cage area.

12. Abdomen: Slide the hands down to the abdomen area.

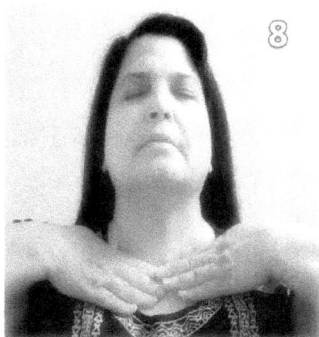

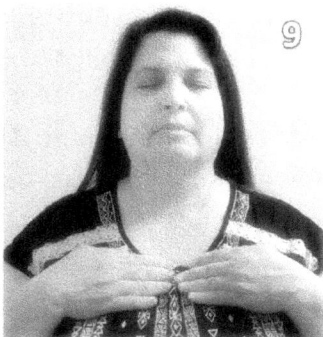

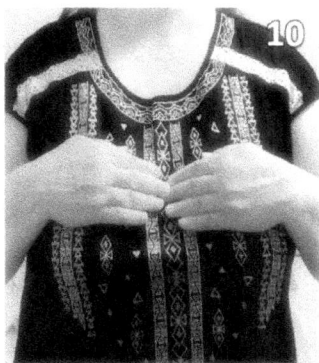

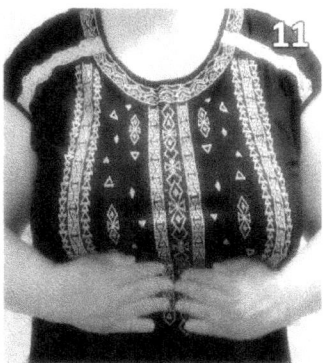

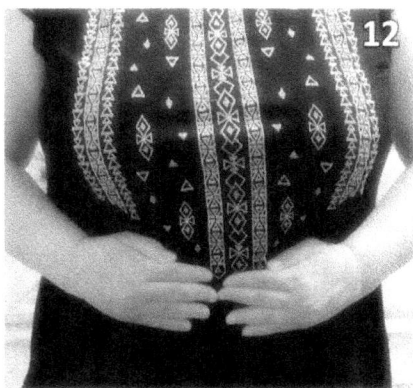

13. Navel (Belly Button): Slide the hands down so the middle finger is aligned with the belly button.

14. Lower Abdomen: Slide the hands down to the lower abdomen (area below the navel and above the pubic bone).

15. Iliopsoas Muscle Area (Crease Where Torso Ends and Leg Starts): Slide the hands down, placing each hand over the crease where the torso ends and the front of the leg starts, with the fingertips pointing toward the pubic bone. This helps with grounding and keeping the energies moving. Maruti Seidman, my Polarity Balancing teacher, taught that old energy can get stuck in this area.

BACK
If you are lying down or reaching toward the back is difficult, you can stay longer on the Abdomen, Navel, and Lower Abdomen positions and skip the back positions.

16. Middle Back: Place the hands on the middle back with fingers pointing toward the centerline.

17. Sacrum: Place the hands in a V form on the lower back with the fingertips over the sacrum.

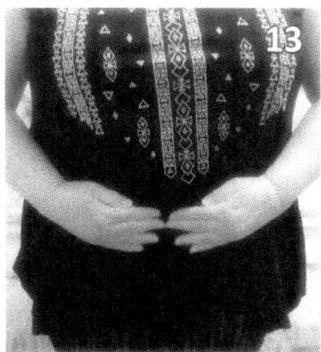
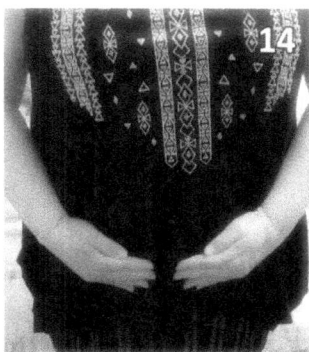
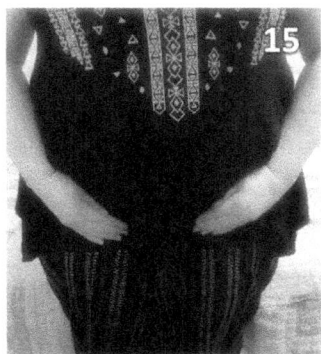
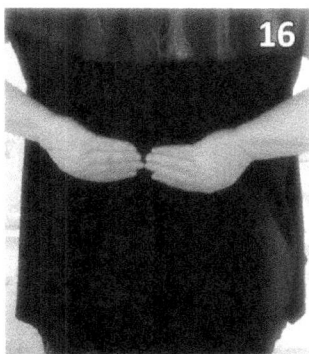
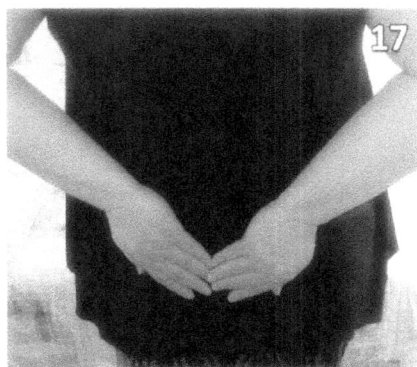

LEGS and HIPS

18. Hips: Place one hand on each hip.

19. Upper Thighs: Place a hand on top of each thigh. If you are lying flat on your back or reaching down to your knees and feet is difficult, you can stay in this position longer and direct the energy to go down the legs where it needs to go and skip the knees and feet positions.

20. Knees: Place a hand on top of each knee.

21. Feet: Please make sure that you are in a comfortable position while doing Reiki on the feet. Place a hand on top of each foot. Then, place a hand on the sole of each foot. This helps with grounding. Alternative: it can also be done one foot at a time by holding one foot with both hands and then switching to the other foot.

For closing, you can do a Connecting Heart and Solar Plexus, followed by tracing a few big 8s with your hands about eight to 12 inches above the torso.

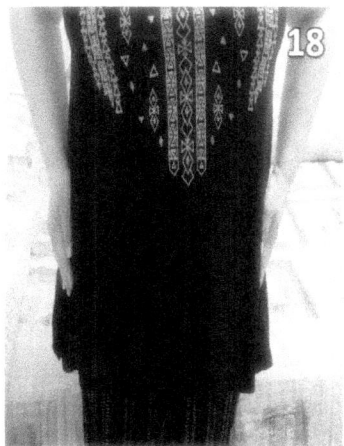
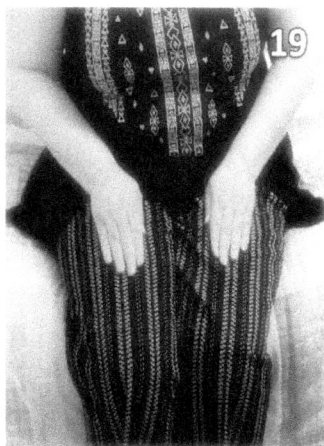
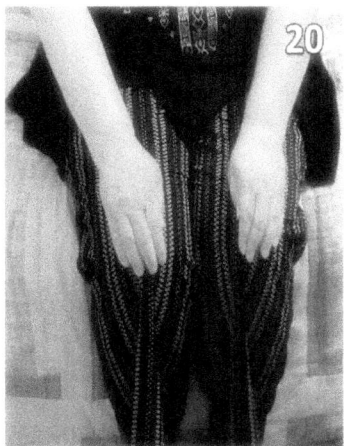
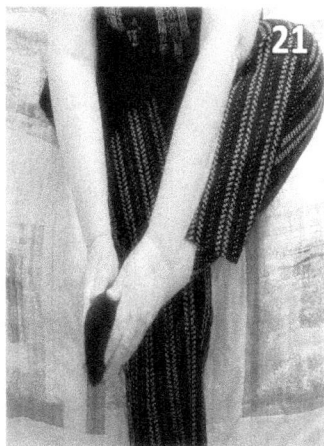

Six

Giving Reiki to Loved Ones

Following are several recommended hand positions for giving Reiki to loved ones. Stay in each position for about two to three minutes (or for as long as you feel it is needed).

Remember:
---Both of you should be comfortable
---Center yourself and set the intention
---Relaxed hands
---Use the Reiki symbols as you feel guided

When the person receiving Reiki is lying down on the back
HEAD
When doing Reiki on the head, it is recommended to position yourself facing the top of the head of the person.

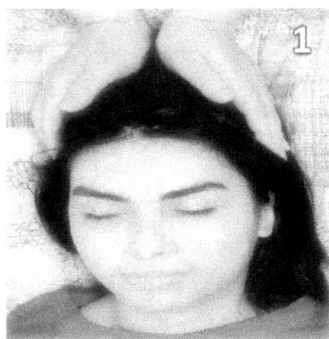
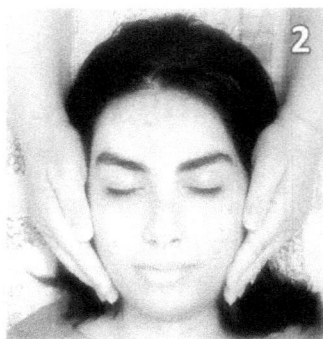
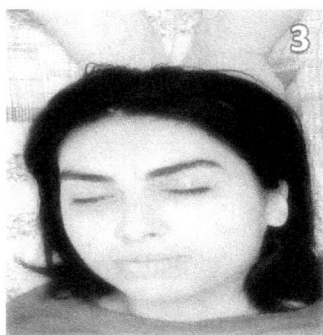
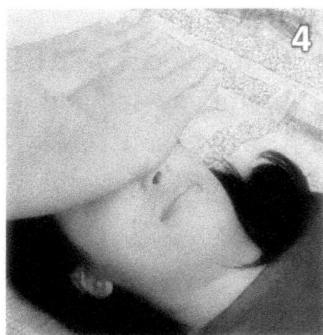
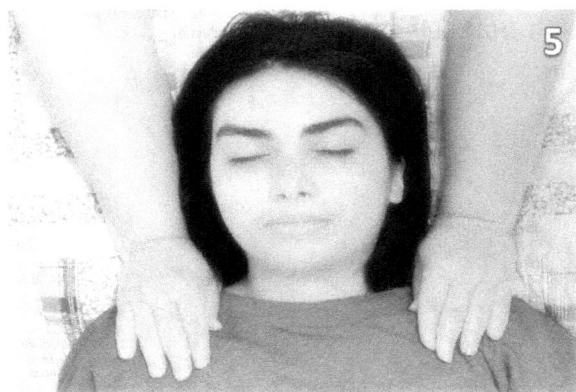

1. Top of the Head: Cover the top of the head by placing the hands with the bottom of the palms touching at the midline of the head and fingertips toward the ears.

2. Sides of the Head: Then, slide the hands down to cover the ears. The fingertips would be resting on the ends of the jaw.

If it is hard to reach the back of the head, then you can hold your hands on the sides of the head for a longer period and skip the back-of-the-head position.

3. Back of the Head: If you can easily reach the back of the head, gently slide the hands down and cradle the back of the head.

4. Face and Neck: If the neck or face areas need attention, give Reiki while maintaining hands side by side in the air about six inches above the surface.

5. Shoulders: Place one hand on each shoulder. This is a very relaxing position for the person receiving Reiki, so stay here as long as you think it is needed.

TORSO

You will be covering the torso by sliding the hands down about a palm's width at a time. Line up the hands by placing one hand with the fingertips touching the bottom of the palm of the other hand. It is okay to place one hand with the fingertips at a close distance but not touching the palm of the other hand; the key is to be comfortable. It is recommended to position yourself to the side of the person receiving Reiki and keep repositioning yourself as you move down the side.

6. Clavicle (Collarbone): Place hands on the clavicle on the upper torso area.

7. Upper Chest: Slide the hands down to the upper chest area.

8. Breast: If the breast area needs attention, give Reiki while maintaining hands in the air about 18 inches above the surface.

9. Rib Cage: Place the hands on the rib cage area.

10. Abdomen: Slide the hands down to the abdomen area.

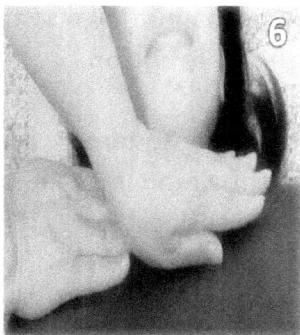

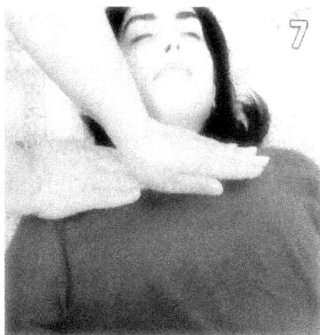

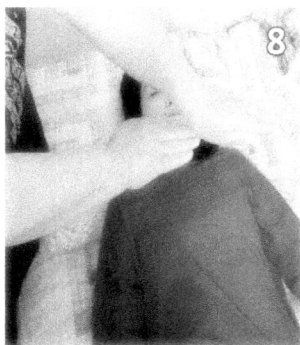

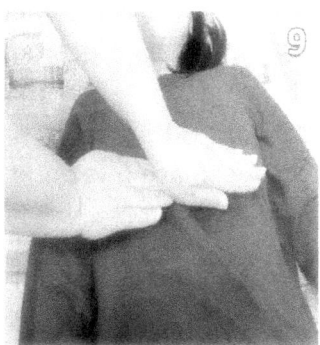

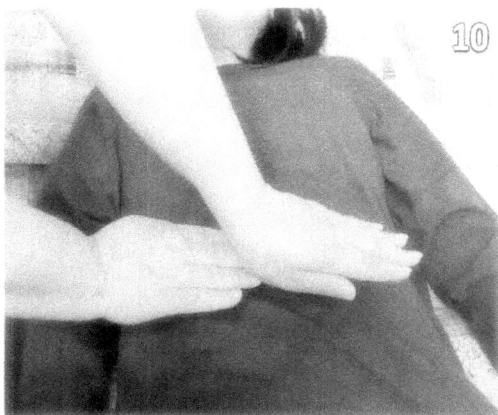

45

11. Navel (Belly Button): Slide the hands down so the middle finger is aligned with the belly button.

12. Lower Abdomen: If the lower abdomen area needs attention, give Reiki while maintaining hands in the air about 18 inches above the surface.

If lying down on the stomach or on the side is difficult for the person receiving Reiki, you can stay longer on the Abdomen, Navel, and Lower Abdomen positions and skip the back positions.

LEGS and HIPS
13. Hips: Place one hand on each hip.

14. Upper Thighs: Place one hand on top of each thigh.

15. Knees: Place one hand on top of each knee.

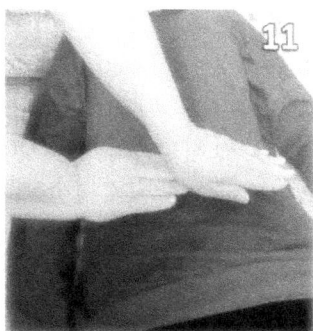
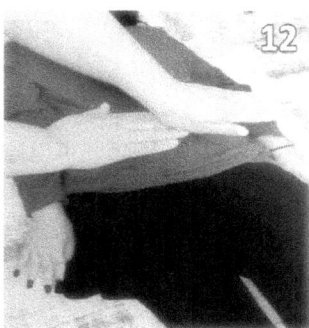
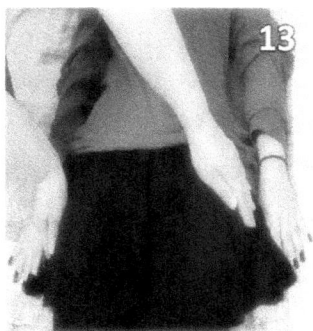
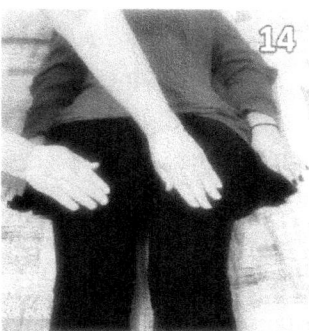
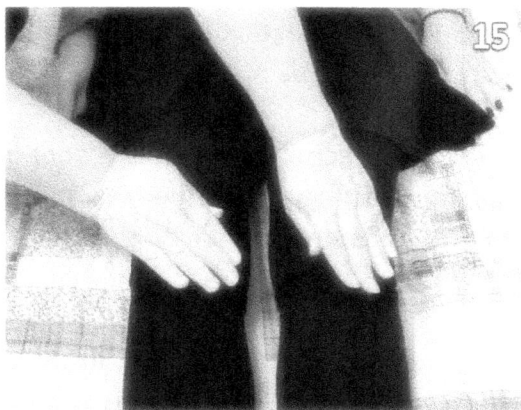

16. Feet: It is recommended to position yourself facing the feet of the person receiving Reiki. Place a hand on top of each foot. Then, place a hand on the sole of each foot. Alternative: it can also be done one foot at a time by holding one foot with both hands and then switching to the other foot.

BACK

If the person is lying down, it is recommended to give Reiki all the way down to the feet while the person is lying on their back before asking them to change positions to lying down on the stomach or on the side for giving Reiki on the back. It is recommended to position yourself to the side of the person receiving Reiki.

17. Upper Back: Place the hands on the line-up position on the upper back.

18. Middle Back: Place the hands on the line-up position on the middle back.

19. Sacrum: If the sacrum area needs attention, give Reiki while maintaining hands side by side in the air about 18 inches above the surface.

Tracing a few big 8s in the air about 18 inches above the person receiving Reiki is a good finishing move when ending a Reiki session.

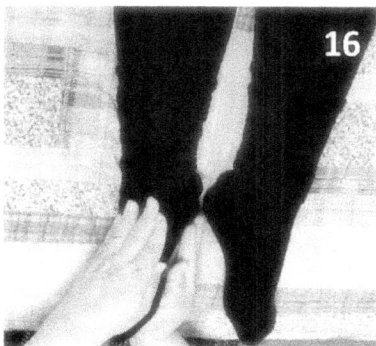

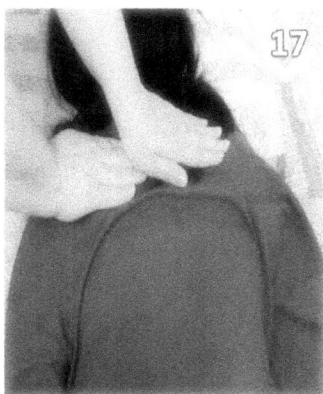

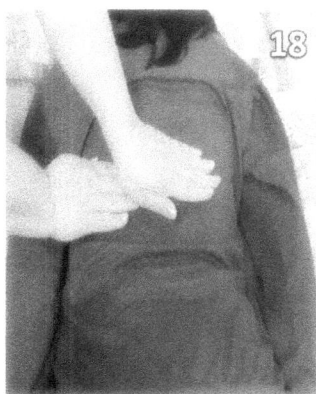

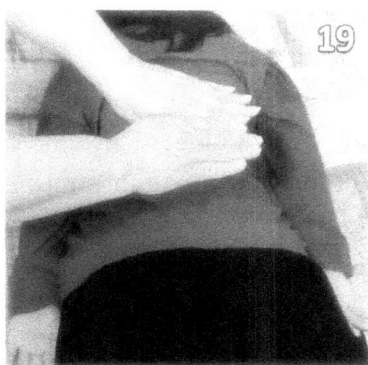

After you finish giving Reiki, it is recommended to trace a few big 8s on yourself and wash your hands.

When the person receiving Reiki is sitting on a chair
If the area needing attention is the head or shoulders, the person receiving Reiki can be sitting on a chair. It is recommended to position yourself behind the person receiving Reiki.

Top of Head: Place your hands on top of the head with fingertips touching at the middle of the crown.

Sides of Head: Slide the hands down to cover the ears.

Back of Head: You can either place the hands on the back of the head sideways or both hands upward.

Shoulders: Place one hand on each shoulder. This is a very relaxing position for the person receiving Reiki, so stay here as long as you think it is needed.

If other areas of the body need attention, while remaining on the shoulders, intend for Reiki to go where needed by saying in your mind:
May Reiki go where it is needed.

Finish by tracing a few big 8s in the air about 18 inches behind the person. After you finish giving Reiki, it is recommended to trace a few big 8s on yourself and wash your hands.

Seven
Archangels

There are many, many, many Angels and Archangels that assist and support humanity. Just as energy can be in different frequencies and have different functions, the Angels have different jobs and work with different frequencies to do their jobs.

Angels do not have physical bodies or gender. They will show themselves to you in the best way for you to perceive them; several of the Archangels pointed this out during our dialogues. Another thing they pointed out is that the Archangels will show themselves in colors different from their traditional color(s).

The Archangels were very supportive. I felt their constant presence while working on this book. The Archangels provided me the information about them that is included in this book during direct dialogues structured in an interview format.

During our dialogues, the Archangels provided information about the meaning of their names, sacred ray they support, their color(s), how can they assist, prayer(s) for assistance, and message to humanity.

Eight of the Archangels stated that they support one of the sacred rays directly; the other Archangels pointed out that they support the sacred rays as needed.

For more information concerning Angels and connecting with them, I recommend:

Connecting with the Angels Made Easy: How to See, Hear and Feel Your Angels by Kyle Gray

The Healing Light of Angels by Raven Keyes

How to Work with Angels by Elizabeth Claire Prophet

How to Be Your Own Genie: Manifesting the Magical Life You Were Born to Live by Radleigh Valentine

The Hall of the Archangels by Radleigh Valentine (online training at: school.radleighvalentine.com/hall-of-archangels)

Archangels 101: How to Connect Closely with Archangels Michael, Raphael, Gabriel, Uriel, and Others for Healing, Protection, and Guidance by Doreen Virtue

Eight
Meet the Archangels

I wrote down the information that was given to me by the Archangels during the dialogues as faithfully as possible. Hopefully this will help you establish a closer connection to the Archangels for when you need to ask for their assistance. Below is the information on the Archangels, in alphabetical order:

Archangel Ariel
"Lioness of God"
The term *lioness* is used to denote bravery.

What is/are your color(s)?
"Red spectrum, from pale pink to red. Red hues. Pink hues. Sparkles. Sparkles that come in any colors. Most people see me in hues in the red spectrum from pale pink to darker. But any color can happen. It depends on the person, how they best would perceive me. But some people see sparkles and rays of light."

Call upon Archangel Ariel:
"Pets, nature, flora, fauna, fairies. Connect with them. Elementals. Connect with nature, fairies, pets. Healing for them."

Recommendations for Prayers for Assistance:

"Dear Archangel Ariel, please help me to better understand nature and connect with the flora and fauna and nature all around."

"They can also say prayers for their pets, like: 'Dear Archangel Ariel, please send healing energies to my pet, (pet's name).'"

Message for Humanity:

"My Dear Ones, Beloved. It is with extreme love and understanding that we assist you upon request. For there is free will; help has to be asked for. So, remember to ask us for help. We will be sure to assist you in any ways we can. For you are very dearest to us. All of you. Blessings. God Bless. Blessings."

Archangel Azrael
"He whom God helps"

What is/are your color(s)?

"People see me in different colors. Mostly in very light colors, like cream, pearly colors. Pearl colors and other light colors. Light blues with sparkles, shiny, iridescent. White light. Pearly light."

Call upon Archangel Azrael:

"For assistance with transitions of life such as transition from career, life stages. Transition from this incarnation. Transitions in many ways. Understand change. To help accept change. That is all for the highest good; that is in Divine Will. To accept that, process and move on to the understanding that it was for the better."

Recommendations for Prayers for Assistance:

"Archangel Azrael, please help me with this change in my life so I accept with grace and understanding that it is all for the highest good. Amen."

Message for Humanity:

"Dear Ones, Beloved. We are all here on this Earth currently experiencing transitions. Lots of turmoil. Lots of change. But please understand that this is for the highest good. After the changes have been accomplished, and like they say, when the waters calm, humanity will be in a better place for the journey toward home. Going back home. Thank you. Blessings. Thank you for your understanding. Blessings to you, my children. For I see you on your way in and on your way out of each incarnation. Blessings again. Until we next meet."

Archangel Chamuel

"The eyes of God" or "He who sees like God"
Archangel of the Third Ray
Third Ray Color: Pink

What is/are your color(s)?

"People see me coming in to them in gold. Golden light. Pale blue. Green; lots of people see me in green. A lot of people see me in pink. But I hold, I support the Pink Ray. I wear, as people see me, mostly green, gold, white. The Light. Manifestations of the Light, of the Rays. People perceive me, mostly green, with some pink. But all colors can happen, too. For I am of the Divine, manifestation of the Divine."

Call upon Archangel Chamuel:

"Love. Joy. Bringing love and joy into their lives. Call upon me for assistance in bringing love and joy into their lives. Self-love and love for others, things, the environment. Divine Love; to bring more Divine Love into their lives. Assistance with pets, their loved ones. If they need assistance with their pets, they can call upon me. Call upon me to help them remember what to do to achieve love, the path taken to Divine Love. So they can love what they create and bring more love and joy into their lives."

Recommendations for Prayers for Assistance:

"Archangel Chamuel, please help me bring joy, happiness, and love into my life."

"Archangel Chamuel, please help me deliver this message of love to my loved one."

Message for Humanity:

"Dear Ones, please remember that love starts from within and grows from your heart out. Love emanates from the heart. So please cultivate the holy flames inside the heart, the Sacred Heart. For they will nurture, replenish. When cultivated, they will bloom to full divinity."

Archangel Gabriel
"For God is my strength"
Archangel of the Fourth Ray
Fourth Ray Color: White

What is/are your color(s)?

"Mix of colors. Copper hues. Whites. Mostly, people see me with the golden halo, copper-hue rim. Copper colors. Copper sparkles. But I come in different colors, for the Light expresses that way. People perceive me the best they can perceive me. Perceive me the best

way for them. Colors... Earth hues, whites, greens, coppers. They perceive me as they wish. That's okay."

Call upon Archangel Gabriel:

"Call upon me to help with communication. To help you achieve your goals. To bring love, happiness, joy, fulfillment into your life. In enterprises, to bring further accomplishments. To help you take care of things you need, I can assist. When you need assistance, call upon me."

Recommendations for Prayers for Assistance:

"Dear Archangel Gabriel, please help me to communicate better in my activities."

"Dear Archangel Gabriel, help me improve my access to creativity."

"Dear Archangel Gabriel, help me with my creative endeavors so I can accomplish my goals successfully."

Message for Humanity:

"Dear Ones, Beloved. Please gather together as the family you all are members of. You are so loved and cared for. Please remember to communicate from the heart. The truth. Always the truth."

Archangel Haniel
"The glory of God" or "The grace of God"

What is/are your color(s)?
"People see me in various colors, shades, hues. But mostly with the colors of very bright light, white light, such as of the moon's. Shades. Silvery blue, iridescent white, and shades of those. Shimmering white light."

Call upon Archangel Haniel:
"They can ask me for many things; I'm always available. Especially for matters dealing with intuition, psychic abilities, natural abilities, and developing them. Women's matters, I can also assist with, and complexities of such. For as you look upon the moon, things that are affected by the moon. Such as emotions, female cycles, and the waves of human emotion. The correlations." (when Archangel Haniel is saying this, I'm seeing in my mind's eye waves in a pool, like ripples; when something starts, and it ripples out)

Recommendations for Prayers for Assistance:
"Dear Archangel Haniel, please help me in developing my intuitive gifts and inner qualities so as to assist me in fulfilling my life purpose and creating a wonderful life."

Message for Humanity:

"Dear Ones, we search for validity in many ways. It is a human characteristic to look for validity. But remember that faith is a true gift. To trust in your inner qualities, abilities. To move forward in your path to achieve your greatness. So have faith in your gifts and trust your guidance. Every day, we give you assistance. We guide you. Especially your Guardian Angels. They guide you. So, listen. Pay attention. Many little things can give messages. A song. A bird. What people call coincidences but are not really coincidences, they are synchronicities. They do carry messages. So, listen. See with your eyes open and you will see that we are always communicating and helping you. And always ask for assistance and we will help more. Because of free will, we can only do certain things to a limit, but with your asking for assistance, we can help you as much as we can, as much as possible. Blessings."

Archangel Jeremiel
"God's mercy"

What is/are your color(s)?

"Shades of purple. People mostly see me in shades of purple. But other colors have been perceived by humans when looking at me. In the shades of purples, reds, hues of pinks, hues of blues, too. But mostly, shades of purple."

Call upon Archangel Jeremiel:

"They can ask for my assistance to awaken their gifts; their special gifts, innately gifts, psychic, intuitive gifts. Help with dream interpretation. Assistance with communicating with Higher Self. Assistance with seeing their path, planning life, seeing the big picture when making plans. I help see the true nature of things and themselves. Also, assist in conveying messages of love."

Recommendations for Prayers for Assistance:

"Dear Archangel Jeremiel, please assist me in seeing clearly my path ahead. What needs to be done in order to achieve my life purpose, my full potential in life."

Message for Humanity:

"Dear Beloved, I welcome you to this reading, to this journey. We of the Angelic Host are very proud of you. For by reading this, you have already taken steps to better connect to the Divine. Please remember to ask us for assistance and we will answer and help you. You are not walking this journey alone. You are never alone. We are here to help you and are walking the path with you all the way."

Archangel Jophiel

"Beauty of God" or "Beholden of God"

(what I get is that it is in the sense of truly seeing God with our hearts)

Archangel of the Second Ray
Second Ray Color: Yellow

What is/are your color(s)?

"I come surrounded in many colors and their many hues. But most people see me coming with colors of yellow, pinks, golds, whites. As you* can see me, I'm coming in with a big halo with colors golden, rim in pink."

*Referring to me during the dialogue, as an example that may apply to others.

Call upon Archangel Jophiel:

"For changing their lives to the most positive way. To seeing the beauty and perspective, seeing the beauty around them. To look into the situation with the wisdom to manifest their lives with more joy and beauty. Divine Beauty, Divine Love. To apply practical knowledge. To obtain the wisdom. Beholding."

Archangel Jophiel is showing me right now something...she moved her right hand and opened it, and sparkles in yellow/gold came out. And she is saying:

"See the magic of life. I can help them see the magic that is truly life. Most people miss that. They get in the routine, in the rut of daily life, and miss that life is magical, so beautiful. Perspective. There is a change in perspective that I can help them with, to see the true nature of how life is, reality is, and how they can change their lives in such positive ways."

"Call upon me if you would like for your life to change to a positive way, the beauty, Divine Love, manifest in your life."

Recommendations for Prayers for Assistance:

"Dear Archangel Jophiel, please help me manifest my life to the fullest beauty and Divine Love."

Message for Humanity:

"Dear Ones, My Beloved. Please remember where you come from and that this life, this experience, is part of your journey. For this has been chosen by you to enrich your soul as you journey back home. There is beauty in life. Much beauty and love."

Archangel Metatron
"He who seats next to God"

What is/are your color(s)?
"People see me in many hues. Deep pinks, deep greens. Shades of green. Shades of pink, to violet, to purples. I also come in blue. Like you* can see me. You* see me in blue. People sense me a little different. Like you* are sensing right now, the pressure on your head versus heat like with most of the other ones. So that is a difference. But in colors, different shades, but mostly in the pink, violet, and green hues."

*Referring to me during the dialogue, as an example that may apply to others.

Call upon Archangel Metatron:
"My children, you can ask me for help with many things. Sincerely, you can ask for many attributes and matters going on in your life. Attributes you would like to develop and matters you would like to correct, resolve in your life. You can ask me for that, you can ask any of us of the Angelic Host. People mostly attribute particular areas, but we can help in all matters as needed."

"For children with special needs, highly sensitive children, you can ask for help to me. You can ask for help for clearing energies that no longer serve you. Stagnant, lower energies. Learning esoteric

knowledge and wisdom. Esoteric matters. Remembering, for most of you, is remembering that wisdom and knowledge from prior incarnations. Call upon me. Time, understanding time. Also, for help warping, stretching time. You can call upon me for knowledge of the geometries, the sacred geometries. You can call upon me."

Recommendations for Prayers for Assistance:

"Dear Archangel Metatron, please assist me in remembering knowledge and wisdom gained in prior incarnations to better help me in this current incarnation."

"Dear Archangel Metatron, please help me heal and clear away any energies that no longer serve me."

"Dear Archangel Metatron, please stretch time to help me get to my destination on time."

Message for Humanity:

"Our children. Behold the new day, for it brings hope of achievement, of new heights, of new skills and knowledge to better equip, to better serve you in fulfilling your life purpose. We love you so much. Please remember to call upon us for assistance and it will be given. Blessings."

Archangel Michael
"He who is like God"
Archangel of the First Ray
First Ray Color: Blue

What is/are your color(s)?
"Sapphire blue, shades of blue, purple, and purple sparkles."

Call upon Archangel Michael:
"Protection and safety; protection in both physical and spiritual. Assistance to reach a destination safely. Seeing things well. Assistance with courage, building confidence, self-confidence, and when having self-doubt. Help with being practical; keeping a practical mind. Help in making things happen. Help in attaining a goal that feels unreachable. Help with building your life, physical things and mechanical things."

"Call upon me for help in many ways. Help with fixing things. Organizing things. Building things. Arranging things. Getting together, camaraderie. Diligently working together toward a common cause. Achieving goals. Creating together. Call upon me to help the world be a better place."

"Call upon me for help. A simple call like 'Archangel Michael, help me' will work."

Recommendations for Prayers for Assistance:

"Dear Archangel Michael, please support me with your angels, so I feel and can be protected and safe."

"Dear Archangel Michael, please surround me, my loved ones, and my home with your beautiful blue light so we are all protected and safe. Amen."

"Dear Archangel Michael, please help me with (explain the situation or what you want to achieve or protection)."

Message for Humanity:
October 2020

My Children,

Please listen to your heart and follow truthfully to make it a reality. Whereas love is paramount and selfish acts are long gone for a shiny, bright future for humanity.

Call upon me when you feel you need courage, confidence, and protection, and it will be answered. Call upon me and my Angels, and it shall be answered. You are much loved. Blessings.

In Love and Light,
Yours truly,
Archangel Michael

November 2020

"We are all so proud of you. We wish you the best. For humanity is working on a journey toward achieving wisdom as they evolve to their true potential. Don't be disheartened. Remember who you are. Remember where your true home is. We love you very much."

Archangel Raguel
"Friend of God"

What is/are your color(s)?

"Shades of blue. People see me in shades of blue."

Call upon Archangel Raguel:

"Relationships. Relationships in many levels. Relationships with each other, like family, romantic. But also, at an expanded level, community, social level. Help to maintain harmony in those relationships and understand when disruption happens, to understand and to heal. Understand the cause of the disruption, misunderstanding, and help heal through forgiveness and peace. If seeking for friends that treat you with respect and wellness, you can call upon me for assistance to attract good relationships, good people into your life that can help you grow and be happy. I also can assist with relationship with yourself, how you see yourself, how you understand yourself, to be true to yourself. That is another level of

relationship that you can ask for assistance with and I will assist."

Recommendations for Prayers for Assistance:

"Dear Archangel Raguel, please help me attract beautiful friendships, harmonious relationships into my life."

"Dear Archangel Raguel, please help me see with clarity this situation with (person's name). Please help me understand so I can take the best path toward healing this relationship."

"Dear Archangel Raguel, please fill my life with wonderful people who love me, respect me, and want the best for me."

Message for Humanity:

"Dear Ones, Beloved. Please remember that we are all one. And relationships with others are relationships with yourself. The Oneself. For we are all together in this journey home. Journey home."

Archangel Raphael

"God heals"
Archangel of the Fifth Ray
Fifth Ray Color: Green

What is/are your color(s)?
"People see me with green hues. Green with gold light around me. Different tones of green. Like emeralds, malachite, and even lighter stones, like prehnite. Shades of green, beautiful green."

Call upon Archangel Raphael:
"They can ask me for help with healing for themselves and loved ones. Help with healing the Earth and Earth's environment. Healing for others (including pets) and self-healing in all the layers. Physical but also emotional and mental. People mostly ask for physical, but I also can help with the other ones."

Recommendations for Prayers for Assistance:
"Dear Archangel Raphael, please send your loving green light to help me heal."

"Dear Archangel Raphael, please send your loving green light to help heal my loved one, (name)."*
*Including pets.

"Dear Archangel Raphael, please surround me and my loved ones with your beautiful green light so we are healthy and well."

Message for Humanity:

"Dear Ones, Beloved. Ask for assistance to help heal the Earth and humanity. Please remember that we are all one, and as one, we move forward to the yonder wishes, to the path. We move in the path together as a family."

Archangel Raziel
"The magic of God" or "Secrets of God"

The term *secrets* is used to denote the magic.

What is/are your color(s)?

"Most people see me in spectrum. Like the light spectrum divided by a raindrop, quartz. Remember rainbows. People see me like rainbows. Reflection of the magic. Rainbows."

Call upon Archangel Raziel:

"They can ask me for assistance, with wisdom, the knowledge, the magical. For there is magic in life, in everything. If you see with your eyes fully open, you will see the magic inherent in life. For doubting, despair, hurt, fears, sorrows, bring the illusion of an ugly reality, personal reality. But if they ask for help, I can assist them in understanding the realities and inherent wisdom obtained with the understanding. For those studying esoteric teachings, that is one of the areas that I can be of assistance with."

Recommendations for Prayers for Assistance:

"Dear Archangel Raziel, please help me gain a deeper understanding of the esoteric information. Please teach me on those areas and help me gain wisdom to guide my life to a better life and deeper understanding of my life purpose and what needs to get done."

Message for Humanity:

"Dear Ones, Beloved. Please seek for my assistance when looking for a deeper understanding of the Universe, reality, and putting that knowledge into wisdom for use in guiding your life and creating a great, optimum reality."

Archangel Sandalphon
"Brother"

What is/are your color(s)?

"People see me as best they can perceive. That is why they perceive me in many colors. Hues between green and blue. Turquoise, soft turquoise. But most people perceive me in the range from the greens to blues."

Call upon Archangel Sandalphon:

"They can ask me for help to deliver messages, their prayers to heaven, and deliver the answers to their prayers. They also can call upon me for assistance with musical notes, in developing music. If you want

to connect, establish connection, and develop yourself with help of the Divine, your inner gifts, spiritual gifts, I can assist. But remember to ask for assistance in delivering your prayers, and I will be there to do so, for it is my pleasure helping."

Recommendations for Prayers for Assistance:

"Dear Archangel Sandalphon, please deliver my prayers to Heaven and bring back the answers to my prayers."

Message for Humanity:

"Dear Ones, Beloved. Seek my assistance and other Angels' assistance. It is not an encumbrance. It is not a chore. It is not a bother. We love you. So, ask for our assistance and we will help you. Again, it is not a bother. We are many, many, many. And we are here supporting you as much as we can. But with free will, it is limited to certain things. So, remember to ask for assistance and we will answer your request for assistance. We love you very much. Blessings."

Archangel Uriel
"The light of God" or "The flame of God"
Archangel of the Sixth Ray
Sixth Ray Color: Purple and Gold

What is/are your color(s)?

"Golden glitter. Purple hues. Ruby sparkles. Bright golden."

Call upon Archangel Uriel:

"They can call upon me for messages to the Divine. Communication with others in a dignified and loving way. Dignity of all aspects of life, of knowing yourself and others. Illuminating your path. For clearly seeing what needs to be done. Expressing your love, your truth. Emotional healing, for it comes from learning your inner truth and accepting it and taking responsibility for your actions."

Recommendations for Prayers for Assistance:

"Dear Archangel Uriel, please clearly show me the way and how best to express myself and relate with others to create a fulfilling and beautiful life."

Message for Humanity:

"Dear Ones, remember who you are. Remember where you come from. Please ask for assistance from any of the Archangels. We all love you. We will assist. But please remember to ask for help, for there is freedom of will. Free will. So, remember to ask and we will answer."

Archangel Uzziel

"The strength of God"
Archangel of the Eighth Ray
Eighth Ray Color: Pink and gold blended into peach hues

What is/are your color(s)?

"People will see me in goldens, pinks, and as a blended peach but also with other colors. Pale greens, pale blues, whites, and a lot of sparkles, golden, silvery. Lots of sparkles."

Call upon Archangel Uzziel:

"For freedom. They can call upon me when they want to be free of ties—self-imposed or imposed by others in their lives. To liberate themselves from what is holding them back from achieving their goals. To free themselves from baggage they're carrying in the ways of emotional and mental burdens, traumas, ways of thinking that do not serve them anymore. Beliefs that do not serve them anymore. To help them reach their full potential, they can call upon me. I'll be there."

Recommendations for Prayers for Assistance:

"Dear Archangel Uzziel, please help me achieve my full potential. Help me let go and free myself of any

binds or ways of thinking or feeling that impede my progress to achieve my full potential."

Message for Humanity:
"Beloved, it is with great pleasure that we provide assistance to humanity to achieve their full potential in their evolution. We love you very much. Please remember to ask us for help and we will assist. We are here in Love and Light. Blessings."

Archangel Zadkiel
"Righteousness of God"
Archangel of the Seventh Ray
Seventh Ray Color: Violet

What is/are your color(s)?
"Purples. People perceive me in hues of purple. Though I come from the Divine Light. Purples, hues of purples."

Call upon Archangel Zadkiel:
"Memory. They can ask for me to help them remember. Also, to help them transform their lives for better; find happiness, peace, and joy."

Recommendations for Prayers for Assistance:

"Dear Archangel Zadkiel, please help me build a fulfilling life full of love, joy, and happiness. Help me take all the steps necessary to make it so, transforming my life to make it such."

Message for Humanity:

"Dear Ones, life is a glimpse. Blip. It is short. Incarnate experience is short compared to the Soul experience. Remember your Soul is having an incarnate experience. And as such, through its path bringing forth love, joy, and happiness. Follow the true path, and so it shall be. Let your heart lead you and ask for help. We are all available. Ask for help and we will assist. You can give us all your fears, worries, and concerns. Ask for help to reach your goals of manifesting a life full of joy, love, and happiness."

Nine
Attunement

Traditionally, the Reiki attunement is given by a Reiki Master Teacher to the student in person. Through the great love these heavenly beings have for humanity, a special dispensation has been granted to allow for Archangels to do the Reiki attunement. Several Archangels have lovingly agreed to provide Reiki attunements.

After reading this book completely, you can petition for an attunement by an Archangel. You can choose any of the Archangels on the list. The attunement is very gentle and will be provided while you sleep after you do the petition.

The attunement will reconnect the person with the Universal Energy, and the person will be able to do Reiki for self and loved ones. During the attunement process, the body and the hand chakras are attuned so the Universal Energy can better flow through them. The Reiki symbols are also activated.

The first thing I felt after receiving my first Reiki attunement was the chakras on my hands. They were warm and pulsing, and I could feel the energy moving.

There are different ways to perceive energy. The key is figuring out what yours are. Some feel energy as heat/warmth or cold, like electricity, as pressure, or as a combination of these.

I mostly feel energy as warmth, sometimes as pressure, and very seldom as electricity.

Ten
Petition for Attunement

Since there is free will, you have to ask for the attunement. After reading this book completely, you can petition for a Reiki attunement by an Archangel. You can choose any of the Archangels on the list:

1.   Archangel Ariel
2.   Archangel Azrael
3.   Archangel Chamuel
4.   Archangel Gabriel
5.   Archangel Haniel
6.   Archangel Jeremiel
7.   Archangel Jophiel
8.   Archangel Metatron
9.   Archangel Michael
10.   Archangel Raguel
11.   Archangel Raphael
12.   Archangel Raziel
13.   Archangel Sandalphon
14.   Archangel Uriel
15.   Archangel Uzziel
16.   Archangel Zadkiel

You can only petition one attunement at a time. You can petition as many times as you want as long as you allow a 21-day cycle for each attunement at a minimum and you read the book completely each time you do a petition. You can petition an attunement each time from the same Archangel or from a different Archangel. Your choice. Each new attunement by an Archangel will enable a stronger connection to the Universal Energy.

Example: I read the book completely and I petition a Reiki attunement from Archangel Michael. This will be day one. Then, on day 22, I read the book again completely, and afterward, I petition a Reiki attunement from Archangel Gabriel.

Following is the Petition for Reiki Attunement. You can say it out loud or in your mind. In the case that the book is listened to instead of being read, please replace "I have read" with "I have listened to" when doing the Petition for Reiki Attunement.

Petition for Reiki Attunement
Dear Archangel *(name)*,
This is *(your name)*.
I have read the *Learning Reiki is Easy* book completely.
I ask you to please bestow upon me the Reiki Attunement.
Thank you. Thank you. Thank you.

Eleven
Give Five

If you believe that this book has helped you:

Please give five minutes of Reiki to Mother Earth and Humanity each day. This will help you practice using the Time/Space symbol to send distance Reiki and will help the world. A win-win.

Please give five dollars to Medical Reiki Works at: medicalreikiworks.org
Medical Reiki Works supports Reiki research and education in healthcare. Medical Reiki Works is a nonprofit organization, so your donation is tax deductible. Another win-win.

I listened to the beautiful songs of the Coqui as I worked on this book. I feel that the songs of the Coqui warm the heart and nurture the soul.

Blessed is one who can hear the Coquis sing at night,
For it warms the heart and nurtures the soul.

Twelve
Recommended Resources

For more information concerning Reiki, I recommend:
The Healing Power of Reiki by Raven Keyes

Sacred Path of Reiki: Healing as a Spiritual Discipline by Katalin Koda

Reiki Fire: New Information about the Origins of the Reiki Power: A Complete Manual by Frank Arjava Petter

Reiki: The Healing Touch: First and Second Degree Manual by William Lee Rand

For more information on the subtle energy body, I recommend:
The Awakened Aura by Kala Ambrose

The Subtle Energy: An Encyclopedia of Your Energetic Anatomy by Cyndi Dale

Energy Medicine by Donna Eden

Balancing the Chakras by Maruti Seidman

For more information concerning Angels and connecting with them, I recommend:

Connecting with the Angels Made Easy: How to See, Hear and Feel Your Angels by Kyle Gray

The Healing Light of Angels by Raven Keyes

How to Work with Angels by Elizabeth Claire Prophet

How to Be Your Own Genie: Manifesting the Magical Life You Were Born to Live by Radleigh Valentine

The Hall of the Archangels by Radleigh Valentine (online training at: school.radleighvalentine.com/hall-of-archangels)

Archangels 101: How to Connect Closely with Archangels Michael, Raphael, Gabriel, Uriel, and Others for Healing, Protection, and Guidance by Doreen Virtue

About the Author

MA Rivera is an energy worker, teacher, and spiritual practitioner. She is a Certified Medical Reiki Master and Reiki Master Teacher who has provided Reiki in private practice and in the hospital setting (including oncology). Through her spiritual practice and empathic nature, she developed a rapport with the Angelic Host and Ascended Masters, which she has maintained for several years. She is passionate about working with the Angels and Ascended Masters to support healing and personal growth.